Baby Massage

Describes techniques of massage that will enhance a child's well-being and maintain the continuity of the bonding process for the mother and father.

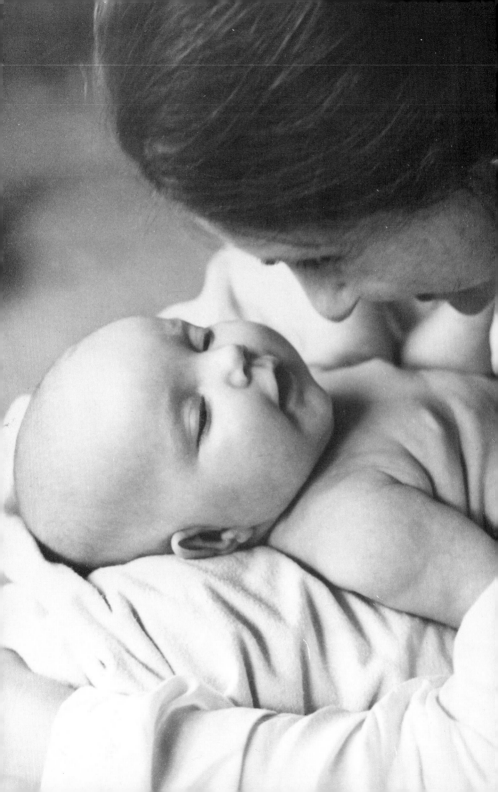

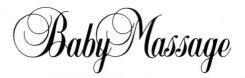

Baby Massage

The Magic of the
Loving Touch

by

Amelia D Auckett

THORSONS PUBLISHERS LIMITED
Wellingborough, Northamptonshire

First published in the United Kingdom 1982

Original Australian edition by
Hill of Content Publishing Company Pty. Ltd.,
Melbourne

Design and photographs by Csaba Banki
Family photographed: Ken, Paola and Bianca Mellor
Line drawings by Rhyllis Plant

British Library Cataloguing in Publication Data

Auckett, Amelia
  Baby massage.
  1. Infants—Care and hygiene
  2. Massage
  I. Title
  649'.4   RJ101
  ISBN 0-7225-0776-3

Printed in Great Britain by
Nene Litho, Earls Barton, Northamptonshire,
and bound by Woolnough Bookbinding,
Wellingborough, Northamptonshire.

Contents

Foreword

Amelia Auckett has written a very important book. It is important as an impetus towards a new age in which humanity regains the capacity for touch, and bodily intimacy from birth, with fellow beings on the planet Earth. Touch is love actualised — through hands, through skin, through genitals, through all the organs of feeling.

The pendulum is reversing. No longer do we consider the body sinful — to be repressed, denied. We humans begin to 'own' our own bodies again. That we own the body is good. I believe God created it from head to toe, from skin surface to the mucous lining of the gut, from lips to genitals. We are no longer as fearful of our nudity; we no longer prohibit our children as much from the exploration of their body surfaces — of themselves, of others. We are more accepting of the pleasure of the feeling flow, which is our birthright, the well of bubbling, joyous aliveness in the here and now.

Flickering like the Aurora Australis (Borealis) in the night sky, our life energy aura responds, luminates and moves under the field of energy emanating from the palm of another who touches. Touch can re-connect longitudinally from head to foot, the broken segments of our life energy flow across cramping barriers. A lump in the throat dissolves as a tender mother strokes her child from face to chest; a spastic diaphragm of a colicky baby relaxes and the lowest rib no longer retracts under the light butterfly stroke from the chest to belly.

Touch was present all around the fetus as the warm uterine wall, buffered by amniotic fluid and lined by a smooth amniotic membrane, continuously rocked the unborn. Natural birth was experienced as a titanic, intermittent 'being squeezed'. The experience of emerging into the new world of air and light, into separate existence, may have been overwhelming. Whatever the experience, the memory of birth and neo-natal life is retained in the 'memory cassettes' into adulthood.

The 'natural law' requires that babies remain bonded to mothers (and vice versa) physically and energetically in the post-natal period. This is achieved primarily by being close, skin to skin. To separate babies and mothers post-partum is a crime against humanity, for thus one ruptures the connection between the energy fields surrounding these two organisms and so interferes with the development or maintenance of the babies' life-supporting link.

The objective reality of energy fields is demonstrated by Kirlian photography, which shows that living bodies are surrounded by an energy field which extends **beyond** the limits of the skin.

The baby massage described by Amelia Auckett in this book can repair the hurt after a difficult birth experience. It can re-bond the ruptured relationships of the family members by re-connecting the energy fields; it can promote natural growth in the untraumatised and traumatised alike.

The beginning of life is the foundation of the whole life time. Those who receive enough touch early, like well-watered and tended seedlings, have a chance to thrive and grow into healthy plants. Separated babies become cold, pale, under-nourished — they sustain a contraction of the life energy field, which can last a life time. Touch can reverse this energetic contraction and stimulate energetic expansion; the pale baby can suddenly become pink, rosy and glowing with sweet warmth.

Loving touch is nurturing, normal. We are not 'spoiling' the baby by using it. Good parenting involves early nurturing, with later release to autonomy and independence. Touch is a precious gift. It is a gift which has value only in the glad acceptance, so it should never be forced on the unwilling. Nor should it be only mechanically applied; and the more delicate the touch, the more delicious is the inner perception in the receiving person, young or old.

Always be responsive to the baby. When the baby has had enough, stop. Touch in baby quantities, delicately and rather briefly, and be sensitive to special needs; if you start in the new-born period, skip over the umbilicus and do not touch it until completely healed.

Touch is natural mammalian behaviour. We must return to this behaviour if we want to become fully human; for touch is a corner-stone of humanism.

Eva Reich[*],
Hancock, Maine, U.S.A.

[*]Eva Reich is a natural childbirth educationist and group therapist. She draws on her experience as a mother, as a Doctor of Medicine in rural, private practice and in assisting home deliveries, as well as a paediatric resident at Harlem Hospital, New York. She is the eldest daughter of Wilhelm Reich, emphasises his concept of self-regulation in her teaching, and uses Medical Orgone Therapy in her group and individual therapy work. She has been an activist in relation to the benefits of birth control, natural childbirth and baby massage, and is in the vanguard of those spreading these ideas around the globe. Countries visited include England, France, Belgium, Holland, Spain, Brazil and Australia.

Acknowledgements

There are many people who have contributed their energies and time to this book, so to all the loving friends who have helped, I wish to express my sincere thanks.

In particular the following have provided both tangible and intangible help which I gratefully acknowledge. They are mentioned in alphabetical order:

Dr David Bannister for support, encouragement, manuscript readings and quotable correspondence; Penelope Goward for reading and commenting on the manuscript; Ralph Hadden for work with early drafts of some chapters; many mothers and babies for their involvement; Ken Mellor for many readings, a large contribution in one chapter, help with editing, suggestions and general support; Barbara Robb for several readings and helpful creative suggestions and Rick Webb for help with typing, editing, ideas, index and support and nurturing.

I give special thanks to my teenage sons Paul and John for their co-operation and for their caring and interest in my book.

Illustrations

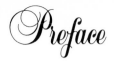

Preface

In November, 1979, I wrote the article, 'Baby Massage: An Alternative to Drugs' for the **Australian Nurses Journal** (Vol. 9, No. 5). It had such wide response from parents and professional people from all around Australia, most of them wanting more information, that I decided to write a book.

My interest in the subject began after I became aware of the baby massage work being done at the Mothers and Babies Health Association Hospital in Adelaide, Australia. There, in August, 1977, I met and talked with Jacqui Showell, a physiotherapist at the hospital. Soon after my return from Adelaide, I introduced baby massage at my Infant Welfare Centre, and now hold regular demonstrations and practice sessions for mothers as well as for Infant Welfare nurses and other Child Care professionals.

I have attended a number of baby massage workshops, including Eva Reich's. The adult massage course I undertook with Terry Suckling, a professional masseur and natural therapist, proved invaluable to me in understanding about massage through experiencing it, and being able to teach baby massage effectively. Also, I have learned a lot about baby massage from the babies I have massaged and have continued to see at regular intervals until they reach three or four years old. The mothers give me interesting and valuable feed-back on their babies' responses and their own responses to the massage.

In 1979, I decided to ask Terry Suckling to work with me, as I wanted to include fathers in baby massage. Terry's massage techniques are compatible with baby massage and can be incorporated with family massage.

We continue to hold Family – Baby Massage Workshops at weekends. Each family includes parent/s and baby. After we talk about massage, I demonstrate the massage on one of the babies. The parents then massage their babies with supervision. We usually have six babies at these workshops. After this, the parents and professional people taking part in the workshops can each experience a head and shoulder massage. As one father said: 'This has allowed me to understand what the baby experiences'. It also teaches parents how to give and receive nuturing. Family massage incorporates a positive interaction of the whole family through a shared learning experience, resulting in improved communication, enjoyment, relaxation, awareness and honesty.

I think it valuable for people who want to teach baby massage to learn about massage through experiencing it themselves. I have found this an exciting and rewarding way to teach parents and others the value of baby massage.

I believe in the effectiveness of baby massage, and I want to share what I have learned with mothers, fathers and people who work professionally with infants and families. I hope, after having read this book, you will **want** to massage your baby, and that you **will** massage your baby and gain as much pleasure and satisfaction from practising the art of massage as I have gained from writing about it.

The ancient art of massage is enjoying a rebirth throughout the world, and it is my hope that this book will make available new ways for people to love and care for themselves and their families. I have included many references to birth, bonding and body contact, because these subjects are all associated with baby massage. It should be noted that I have used 'he', 'him' and 'his' in the text simply to distinguish the baby from the mother.

'Nurturing for Parents' is included as a special chapter because, if nurtured themselves, parents can better care for their children.

Amelia Auckett,
Melbourne
September, 1981

Birth and Bonding

Experience this with me:

I'm a very little person.
I'm completely surrounded, supported, nourished,
    warmed, cushioned
Swimming in a warm sea
I am one with my mother
At one with my newness
Feeling, hearing a heart beating, blood rhythmically
    surging around me, feeling safe and warm.
There is movement, this way and that
I am one with my mother's feelings; I feel it too
    when she is angry, sad, loving, happy.
With my mother, I experience other people, hear their
    muted sounds, feel their touch.
I am very small, surrounded by a supporting,
    nourishing, vast, loving universe.

As I steadily grow
My limbs stretch and flex
Against the soft boundaries of my world
And my back is caressed.
Then gradually my space becomes crowded,
I curl up
I curl into a ball
I feel confined, cramped
I long to stretch
To be free!
Then, dawning joy,
Rhythmical pulsations press me
And caress my skin,
Becoming stronger
As I start moving down a narrow tunnel.
Strong emotions and sensations
Surge through me.
It's time to be born!
Time to leave the warm womb
Time to experience my new life
The strong pressure eases

As I emerge —
I am free!

Gentle hands lift me onto
My mother's smooth skin,
We lie belly to belly
I feel her warmth
I hear again the familiar rhythm
Of her heartbeat.
I open my mouth
I cry once, then again,
As air fills my lungs
Then I breathe strongly.
Nuzzling her breast
My face pressed to her,
I find the nipple
Warm food flows into my mouth as I suckle.

Then I feel her stroking my head
And body — my back, my limbs.
My cord is cut,
Ending links with the womb,
Yet I feel safe
With our new bond already strong.
Our energies merge in a flow of love
As we look at each other,
As I hear her voice
And I respond to her touch,
Her smell, her taste.

Here, close to mother
I feel safe, nourished, warm
I belong.
I am.

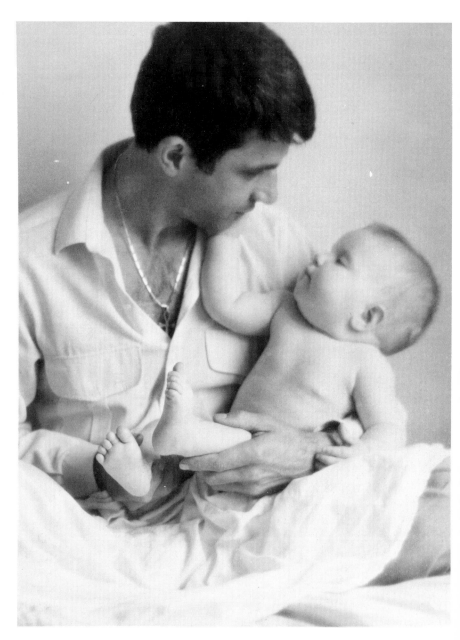

Inside the womb, the baby has a rich sensory input, the sounds of the mother's own body and sounds from the outside world, movement as the mother moves, and a high tactile input with the baby completely surrounded and supported all around by the womb. Every emotion the mother feels has its physiological effect on her body, and the baby, intimately connected to her, experiences these too.

During birth, the baby undergoes an immensely strong, almost overwhelming experience, squeezed by powerful uterine contractions and moved down the narrow birth canal and out into the world.

By being placed gently on the mother's bare belly before the cord is cut, he will feel at peace and secure as he has eye contact with his mother and is caressed by her, and nuzzles and finds her breast. It is interesting to note that the umbilical cord is generally just long enough so that the baby can suckle at the breast. The stimulation from this suckling releases hormones — oxytocin, which stimulates lactation and contracts the mother's uterus, thus assisting in the expulsion of the placenta, and prolactin, the other hormone, which induces the production of breast milk.

In the womb and during the process of birth, the umbilical cord supplies all the oxygen the baby receives, until the baby emerges into the air and takes his first few breaths. At this stage, oxygen comes from these two sources, the cord and the air, and dependence on the umbilical cord ceases only when the special valve in the baby's heart closes so that the pulmonary system takes over for the rest of his life. It is, therefore, important that the cord is cut only when it stops pulsating, so that the changes from womb to world, from depending on the mother, to oxygenating his blood with his own lungs, becomes a smooth transition. This is a beautiful time for all, and is involved in allowing mother and baby the close contact they need while they are physically linked and are making the transition to another form of bond.

This is the moment for massage to begin.
Very lightly. Very lovingly.

Since Frederick Leboyer's book, **Birth Without Violence**, was published in 1974, many parents want to have a 'Leboyer birth' for their baby.[1] This is a gentle birthing process that takes place in great silence with low lighting and gentle, loving hands allowing the baby to learn to breathe before the cutting of the cord; then allowing time for suckling at the breast — and for bonding — before he is given a warm, relaxing bath.

This kind of birth is available in some maternity hospitals around the world, particularly where there is a Birth Centre. However, more parents are deciding on home births of the Leboyer type, where there are minimum medical, technological and nursing procedures to interfere with the normal birth process. Thus the birth experience, the bonding and the welcoming time all belong to the parents and their new baby. The mother and her baby are not separated. They are close together, where they belong, and soon get to know each other; the father at their sides, involved, loving and bonding too, to his new family.

Bonding is the strong physical, emotional and spiritual attachment which can develop between people of any age. Mothers, fathers and babies need a special time together immediately after birth for this attachment to develop. Bonding between parents and their new baby is a very significant event.

The importance of bonding through skin contact and close body contact straight after birth has been carefully described in the book, **Maternal-Infant Bonding**, by M. H. Klaus and J. H. Kennell.[2] They have called this time 'The Maternal Sensitive Period'. I have heard Eva Reich called this

period 'The Welcoming Hour'.

Bonding is developed by the baby through touch, sight, hearing, taste and smell. Behaviour by the mother and father such as fondling, kissing, cuddling and prolonged gazing, are indicators of bonding attachment to their baby.

The ideal birth I have described is not always possible. Sometimes things go wrong and skilled medical help is needed.

Events which interfere with the bonding process are: delay in infant and mother and father being together after birth; drugs which anaesthetise either the mother or the baby or prolonged separation after a Caesarian Section; the necessary use of the Isolette. Massage given to such babies by a person other than the parent can reduce many of the harmful effects of separation. If, when the mother or father is available, she or he massages the baby, this, together with other forms of closeness, such as cuddling, rocking and holding, will reinforce and continue the bonding process. The opportunity for bonding that would otherwise have been lost can thereby be salvaged and the bonds strengthened.

Often the procedure in hospitals during the so-called 'normal' birth involves noise, bright lights, separation from the mother, and little opportunity for bonding. In addition to these insults, the baby has undergone the turbulence of the birth itself, suffered the loss of security he had known in the warm womb, and the shock of finding himself in the isolation and emptiness of the bassinette. He is also denied the nurturing contact he needs. Massage is valuable for these babies too, as it is particularly effective in reducing the consequences of birth trauma.

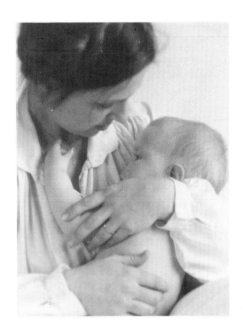

Loving Touch

Massage is an expression of love through a special kind of caring touching. When mothers massage their babies at an early age, the massage continues the bonding process and helps establish a warm, positive, parent-child relationship. It also creates a metaphysical energy flow, which could be called a flow of love between mother and baby. This is an energising experience, and deep communication is possible. Baby massage is an introduction of caring touch to an infant that can continue to any age. Toddlers, teenagers and adults seem to be more receptive to touch if they were massaged as babies. Either parent can massage the baby. However, in what follows I am talking mainly about mothers.

Nutritional Value of Touch

Human touching provides a vital nutriment for the baby. All babies need a balanced diet, including the right vitamins and minerals, and if, for example, the premature baby does not have extra iron added to his feeding, he will develop anaemia, with a consequent set-back to his normal development. With an adequate supply of iron, such a baby follows a normal developmental pattern, and thrives. So it is with loving touching. If there is a lack of this, the baby's emotional and physical development is impaired; if it is given freely, he develops normally, becoming healthy, vigorous and aware.

Massage for the Unsettled Baby

In discussion about baby massage with Dr David Bannister, a Melbourne paediatrician, he had t[h] to say:

> Sometimes mothers and babies don't 'click' or bond automatica[lly] and if the baby is a difficult 'colicky', irritable, non-responsiv[e] baby, then the mother may have difficulty coping, adjusting or understanding her baby, and angry negative feelings can develop. The mother may draw away from her child, rather than towards him, and the interactior around this crying baby may sometimes engender hostile, aggressive feelings. The interjection of a positive, touchir caressing approach may be invaluable in altering the mothe[r] negative reaction to a positive, tender, warm response. This car only be a good thing for mother and baby. I consider baby massage to be beneficial to bab[y] from a very early age. It gives th[e] mother something positive to d[o] for her screaming 'colicky' baby, and if it calms the baby down without the use of drugs, then th[is] is a good thing. I think what you are doing in teaching the mothe[r] to massage their babies is good.

14

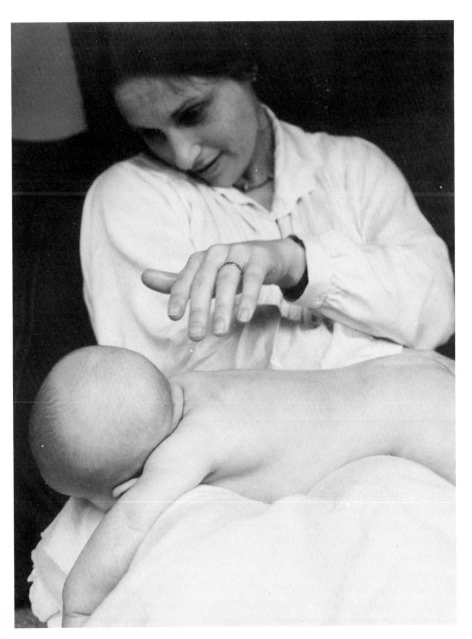

Massage to Reduce Stress

Generally, baby massage is useful in reducing stress between parents and their babies. It is often very useful for mothers (or fathers) who were battered as babies and now find some difficulty in caring for their babies in a gentle, caring, loving way. Through learning to massage, they find that they can give their babies a pleasurable and healing experience through touching. Also a mother (or father) who may be battering his or her own baby, is given an alternative, positive way of interacting, a way that can soothe the baby's crying and distress, and enable both parent and baby to feel happier in themselves and more loving towards each other. I think that baby-battering is often due to unresolved, excessive stress, and I believe that the practice of baby massage can do much to reduce its incidence. Appropriate counselling, medical help or other forms of support may also be needed.

Massage — An Alternative to Drugs

When through massage a warm loving relationship is developed, and a positive flow of love is established between the parents and baby, massage can then become an alternative to drugs. The love of the parent, directly expressed through touch, promotes relaxation, and encourages the baby's growth and self-healing potential. Massage is beneficial to babies in their developing years, and can remain valuable throughout their lives. When early bonding is well established and the mother-child relationship becomes warm and caring, it lays the foundation for similar warmth and caring with others in later life.

Parents' Experiences

I have seen satisfactory results with moderately to severely unsettled babies and moderately to severely anxious mothers. After massage the babies have become smiling and pink and very relaxed, and the mothers have become smiling and happy and have begun to enjoy their babies. The most frequent comment from mothers is, 'It works, and I enjoy it too'. Here are some examples:

> One mother told me how her baby always became excited and his eyes lit up when he realised he was about to have his daily massage, and I feel that this highlights the benefits of daily massage.

> 'Jane' started massaging her baby daily (full body massage) at six weeks of age. The mother appeared more relaxed after the massage commenced. She continued regular massage until the baby was eight months old. At

this age, he was a responsive, active and very aware baby. 'Jane' had commented when her baby was six months old: 'It helped him to learn who I am and that I'm going to be there when he wakes up. I feel more aware of his body shape and the texture of his skin. I've gained a lot of confidence and I'm not scared to touch him; I just know we both like it'. When the baby was eleven months old, she said: 'I occasionally give him a full massage still, and recently when he was teething, I massaged his shoulders and neck. This was very effective in soothing him. I have not given any drugs to my baby in his eleven months of life'.

I see this last statement as most significant. This baby, in fact, has not needed to get sick in order to have his needs met. This mother, with her loving caring touching and close communication, has met her baby's physical and emotional needs. 'Jane' and her husband exchange massages, so that sharing pleasurable touching is a way of life in this family.

'Lois', who massaged her baby from six and a half weeks of age, commented when her baby was four months old: 'I have touched something very delicate. It's beautiful. It's somewhere I haven't been before. I tune in as one — we become one'. This mother was over anxious. Her baby cried a lot and had 'colic'. Merbentryl was given to the baby for four months. This mother had some full body massages from a professional masseur and some back and neck massages from her husband. Through being nurtured in this way, she was able to massage her baby to their mutual satisfaction and pleasure. It gave her something positive to do for her baby and calmed them both.

'Lois' goes on to say: 'My baby is now nineteen months of age, and whenever I run my hands over his body, a pleasurable smile greets me; this, I feel, is a great gift which he has received for life, for he is now a responsive, lovable, affectionate human being in which massage would have played an important role'.

I recently spoke to a group of mothers with toddlers of eighteen months, all of whom had massaged their babies. These toddlers showed a great deal of affection for their mothers and one another, and played happily together. We held the group in the garden of one of the mothers. Instead of clinging to their mothers, these children played with toys, explored the garden and enjoyed themselves. They are very aware, responsive, stable children, and have a lot of self confidence.

These mothers still massage their toddlers from time to time, particularly in times of stress such as teething. One toddler, Nicholas, when he needs some attention, goes to his mother and pulls up his T-shirt indicating that he wants a 'tummy tickle'. Surely this infant has learned to get his needs met in a positive, enjoyable, open way. Each of three of these mothers is expecting a second child, and all three of them are going to massage their babies from birth onwards.

In a questionnaire on baby massage one mother wrote:

> I feel it is important if you want to build a bond with your child. My son refers to his massage as 'a tick a tick'. He asks for it when he's upset; he knows it is something to make the 'feeling' he has disappear. We have a very good communication level which I think is due to massage and body contact. When I started massaging him, we also developed a silent communication with our eyes. He is now able to tell whether or not I'm angry or pleased, through my eyes. I feel our relationship took on a new meaning when we started massaging at about two or three months. My son is nearly two years old now. The relationship is still growing.

Finally, another mother told me:

> I had no trouble in doing the massage, and I started when my baby was two weeks old. He is now twenty-five weeks old. I usually give him three or four full massages a week, then a massage of face and hands whenever I feel like it.

> In the beginning, I massaged for ten minutes, and now take twenty to thirty minutes, unless he indicates that he wants a shorter time.

> During the massage, my baby relaxes, smiles, plays with his own limbs, pats me and tries to talk. Afterwards he is quiet and relaxed and sometimes sleepy. If we do a massage at about 7 p.m., he quite often sleeps longer through the night.

> Apart from when he has wind, constipation or tummy aches, he usually cries only when he is hungry.

> His ability to communicate has developed well, and he is bright and alert. I have quickly learned to recognise by his voice when something is wrong.

> Massaging my baby has made me more confident with him; I am more relaxed and really enjoy this

time together. After massaging the baby, I usually like to give my other son time and attention, and sometimes give him a massage too.

One thing I like is that the older children or their father can give massage to the baby. Communication is improved with massage, and I think it would be especially good for fathers, as they quite often spend so much time away from home. It is particularly good for fathers who have attended their child's birth, to keep the emotional bond going.

No special equipment is needed for baby massage.

I have noticed that my baby is not only aware of his own body, but is more aware of other people.

My husband thinks massage helps to relax the baby and to relieve any tension, and is good for toning up the baby's muscles after he has been lying down for any length of time.

We prefer to use massage instead of medicines to calm him down after he has been upset. Many people have commented on how well-behaved and happy our baby is on outings, and we assume they mean quiet and relaxed. We have always credited this to massage.

Benefits of Baby Massage

For mother or father:

> Pleasure, enjoyment, permission to touch;
> Communication, confidence, gentleness;
> Relaxation, relief from anxiety;
> Oneness with baby;
> Something positive to do for baby;
> Energy sharing between mother, father and baby.

For baby:

> Pleasure, joy;
> Permission to touch and be touched — this will flow on to later life;
> Communication, closeness, gentleness;
> Relaxation and calmness;
> Reassurance through skin contact;
> Better sleep pattern;
> Develops body awareness;
> Breaks the anxiety-pain cycle, improving digestion;
> Improving circulation, increasing resistance to illness;
> Oneness with mother, father;
> Emotional contact;
> Energy sharing between baby and mother, father.

Ashley Montague in his important book, **Touching**[3], says that when certain young animals experience skin stimulation, the immune system benefits, resulting in a positive

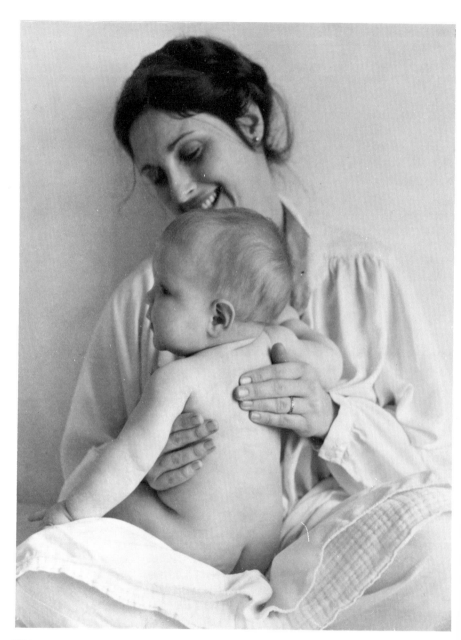

improvement in disease resistance.

He believes it probable that human skin touch can help in the growth of 'healthy emotional or affectional relationships'.

He makes the important observation that being loved, when learning to love, is superior to instruction in loving.

Energy Exchange

Parents and professional people often ask, 'But what do you mean by energising, exchange of energy, and the needs of a baby to get subtle energy from his mother?'

Some babies are jaundiced at birth or soon after, because of a blood problem, and need an exchange transfusion; that is, their blood is gradually removed as they slowly receive completely new blood **from another person**. This allows the baby to survive and live a normal, healthy life. This is a physical exchange.

However, an energy exchange cannot be seen, but it can be felt, and the result can be seen, as illustrated in the following example:

In the family massage workshops that I run with Terry Suckling, there is always a baby that is upset and crying, and doesn't want to be massaged. We suggest to the mother that she has a head and shoulder massage, and within a few minutes of Terry starting the massage on her, the baby calms down, even though he is being held by another person — usually me. By the end of the massage, in about twenty minutes, the baby is in a deep sleep, and usually sleeps for over an hour. This is a positive example of an energy exchange.

Energy exchange is very aptly explained by Jean Liedloff in her book **The Continuum Concept** when describing her experience with the Yequana Indians in Venezuela:

> In the infant kept in constant contact with the body of a caretaker, his energy field becomes one with hers and excess energy can be discharged for both of them, by her activities alone. The infant can remain relaxed, free from accumulating tension, as his extra energy flows into hers.[4]

In the Parenting Workshop which I attended in 1977, Ken Mellor, a Melbourne social worker, talked about ways of handling a frantic screaming baby who is not hungry or sick. He stated that, in his experience, what these babies often needed was **subtle energy from their mothers**. If the mother was depleted, he suggested that she be nurtured in order to foster the flow

21

between herself and her child.

I have held some of these frantic babies and have felt them drawing energy from me.

However, if the baby's need is to discharge energy rather than receive it, going for a brisk walk or dancing around the room with baby in your arms or supported in a sling, will often calm him down, as his energy flows into yours.

It is heartening to see that more parents are becoming aware of the benefits of body contact with their baby, because it promotes this energy exchange.

There is an energy link between the mother and baby which is involved in giving the baby his security. Without this link the baby is very likely to become distressed because he feels cut off from his mother.

This energy bonding is a most important part of mothering.

Parents who massage their babies, expressing their loving caring through touch, experience the flow of love-energy. As this life-energy is allowed to flow in babies and adults, it promotes self-healing, resulting in happier, healthier people.

Close Body Contact
There are other ways of continuing skin contact and close body contact in a loving way as well as through massage. The baby can have a bath with either of the parents. Fathers often enjoy a bath with their new baby. (Japanese parents and children bathe together until the children are about ten years old.) Breast feeding is also an important way that baby can experience skin and close body contact. Bottle feeding while the baby is against bared breast or chest is a variation on this. Some parents are finding that if their baby is unsettled at night, and they take baby into their bed, he settles down with the close body contact and all sleep well. This can be particularly effective if the baby decides to scream at 3 a.m.! Others extend this principle by having their baby sleep with them until some months after the birth.

In our society, babies often spend a great deal of time alone in bassinettes, bouncinettes, prams and carry baskets. Carrying an infant in a baby sling such as the 'Meh Tai', or the 'Joyride', gives the baby much needed body contact. The baby feels the rhythmical movement of his mother's body, hears her voice and heartbeat, and identifies her unique body scent. He feels secure. This is a practical way of caring for the baby and doing house-keeping tasks at the same time, hanging out the washing or doing the shopping.
A baby cannot be 'spoiled' by close body contact.

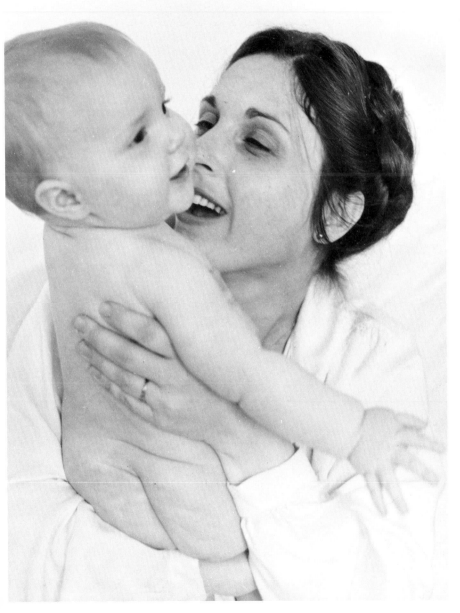

Technique

Summary

Basically, the massage flows from top to toe, simply starting at the head and following on to face, neck, shoulders, arms, chest, belly, legs and feet. To finish the front of the body, use long, light strokes from neck to toe. Then, turning baby on to his belly, you massage his head, neck, back, buttocks, legs and feet. Again, finish with long sweeping strokes from head to toe. The whole massage takes about twenty minutes, or however long you and your baby want to take.

It is important for both adults and babies, that all massage be given in a symmetrical way, that is, on both sides of the body, left and right.

If only the left or the right side of the body is massaged, it can result in a feeling of imbalance with one leg or one arm feeling 'alive and lighter', and the other leg or arm feeling 'heavier' leaving a sensation of being 'unfinished'.

What Kind of Touch for Your Baby?

To begin with, use the lightest feather-touch, and increase the pressure if you sense your baby's need for it. This is because many people (and babies are people) differ in their tolerance to degrees of touch. Your baby will let you know with joy the best touch to use.

Stroke or massage each area of the body described two or three times. On small areas use just the fingertips, for large areas use the fingers and palm. Some parts of the body will be massaged with one hand, other parts with both hands used simultaneously.

In the description to follow, 'stroking' means just sliding lightly along the surface of the skin, 'massaging' means gently moving muscles beneath the skin. Throughout the massage, you can change back and forth from the light flowing stroking to the slightly deeper, localised massaging, but always finish with light strokes so baby will stay relaxed.

Strokes should be flowing and free and need not be restricted exactly to the area described. When stroking the neck, for example, each stroke will naturally flow on to touch the shoulders and upper back, or when stroking down the arm, each stroke will include the fingertips and move beyond them.

It is best to have short fingernails when massaging anyone, but especially babies. If you must have long nails, make sure you use the balls of your fingers and the palms of your hands, and do not scratch baby. At the beginning of the massage, after washing your hands, rub them together until warm.

Is Oil Necessary?

When the light touch is used for baby massage, oil is usually not necessary. When massaging the back, oil can be useful, especially if the mother's hands have become moist.

If you do use oil, I recommend a cold pressed vegetable oil (apricot or almond are suitable), obtainable from most health food stores. A cold pressed vegetable oil will nourish and moisten the skin, feels very smooth and pleasant, and it won't harm baby if he sucks his hand. The daily use of oil is particularly helpful if your baby has very dry skin. In the winter, warm the oil by placing oil bottle in a container of hot water. Do not pour oil directly on to baby's skin, but pour a little oil on your own hand, hold it briefly to allow it to warm or cool to skin temperature, then smooth on to the part of the baby's body which you are about to massage. Do not use oil on the face; it is neither necessary nor pleasant.

For Babies Under Four Weeks

(Including Premature Babies)
Only a short massage, approximately ten minutes.

Light gentle strokes, being aware of sensitive areas. Many young babies, for example, at first don't like being touched on the head (particularly if the head experienced a lot of pressure during birth); also be gentle with the neck if at birth the cord was around the neck. You can accustom the baby to a gentle touch and soothe away the hurt gradually, with each massage, by increasing the length of time you stroke the sensitive area, from a few seconds to a minute or so.

Bath time is a good time to massage young babies, as it eliminates the need to undress and dress the baby an extra time.

Also, with young babies, massage can be done without completely undressing the baby, e.g. the abdomen and legs, while leaving on upper clothes.

Do what the baby enjoys and respond to his needs.

The First Time

I suggest that the first time you massage your baby, you do it only when you and your baby are relaxed and happy and the baby is not hungry. If you do this, then there will be imprinted on the baby's body memory an association of the massage with a relaxed and happy feeling. After the initial association is made, you will later be able to use the massage to soothe and calm your baby when he is upset or distressed.

Should you start feeling upset while doing the massage, just go with the feeling; you are probably experiencing his pain (for example, his birth trauma), or getting in touch with pain you experienced early in life. If the baby becomes upset too, stop and give him a cuddle, as massage should be a pleasurable experience.

Work out a time that suits you both for your baby's daily massage.

Become familiar with as much of the technique as possible before you begin, by reading it through a few times.

There are Two Types of Massage
The first type of massage is for pleasure and fun for both you and your baby; and the second is for sharing, that is, a loving exchange of energies between you and your baby. This flow of love brings a special kind of closeness to you and your baby and allows the life energies to flow. It gives you both an increased feeling of well being. Combine these two types of massage and then, peacefulness, pleasure, fun and a wonderful communication between you and your baby will begin.

Massage is Communication
A great deal of communication takes place through the eyes. So during the massage, be in eye to eye contact with baby as much as possible. Part of flowing communication involves flexibility, so be flexible. If the baby wants to turn around or change position somehow, don't forcibly hold him in position so that you can do that step of the sequence, just massage the part of the body that is accessible to you then, working in the head to toe direction. You can return later to the areas you missed.

You are probably aware that your baby, like an individual, is special and unique and has his own likes and dislikes, including where and how he likes to be touched. He is able to communicate this to you. So listen to, look at and feel what he is saying about his long term dislikes or short term dislikes, for example: 'Today, I don't want my face touched'. In this way, you can discover the strokes that you and your baby most enjoy and develop your own special style of massage which will change according to your baby's needs and growth.

There are some babies who basically have a highly sensitive temperament or low threshold of sensitivity and cannot tolerate too much stimulation for too long. For these babies, begin by giving very gentle, short massages, gradually lengthening the time as their tolerance to loving touch increases. Occasionally a baby may not be responsive to massage, however gentle. If this is so, try increasing close body contact and skin to skin contact in other ways. For example,

26

the baby may be held against the bare chest of the father or mother. Remember that loving, caring touching is needed.

The massage can be poetic, sensual and fun; an art, not just a mechanical technique. As you massage, enjoy feeling the softness of his hair, appreciate the beautiful shape of his arm, talk to your baby, tell him what lovely eyes he has, tell him 'Your skin is just like velvet'.

Preparation
Prepare the room beforehand, so that it will be warm for baby. Turn on the heater or open the drapes allowing the warm sunshine and light to stream into the room. Disconnect the telephone and close the door. Take off your jewellery, remove your shoes. With baby lengthways on your lap, head towards your feet, sit comfortably on a cushion on the floor, with your back supported, or in a bean bag, in the sunlight or in front of the heater or open fire with its golden glow of warmth. Alternatively, place baby on a yoga mat or sheep skin on the floor and kneel beside him. Undress baby completely, but if he seems to be cold, cover parts not being massaged with a bunny rug. Place a towel under baby's bottom and have some nappies at hand, for the sign of a good massage is a good wee.

You are now ready to begin.

The Beginning

This is an important moment.
A loving sharing is going to take
place and this is something special
between you and your baby.
Be calm, be peaceful.
Listen to, look for, and feel the body
language of your baby.
Ask yourself — 'How does he feel
right now?'
Then talk to him.
Tell him how you feel him to be as
you start slowly and gently to stroke
him.

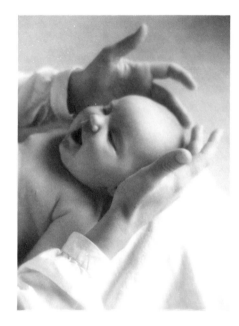

How to Massage your Baby.

The Front of the Body:

The Head:
Stroke the crown of the head with one hand, using a circular movement. Be gentle with, but do not avoid, the fontanelle or 'soft spot'. Then, with the fingertips of **both** hands stroke from the crown of the head down along the sides of the face.

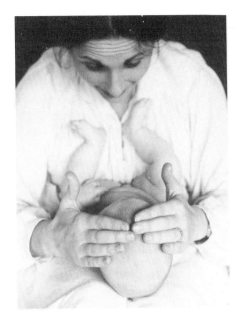

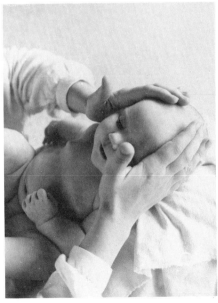

Face:

With the fingertips, lightly stroke the forehead from the centre to the temples, then lightly massage temples using a circular movement. Stroke the eyebrows from nose to temple; the bony ridges below the eyebrow and below the eye to the temple; from the nose, over cheeks to the ears. With fingertips stroke from the corners of the eyes down the sides of the nose to the corners of the mouth; stroke from centre of the chin along the jawbone to the ears. Stroke behind each ear starting at top. Stroke the ears back and front, following the shape of the ears.

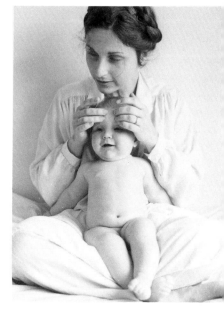

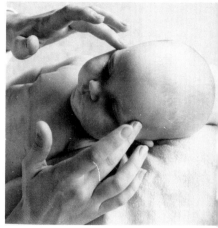

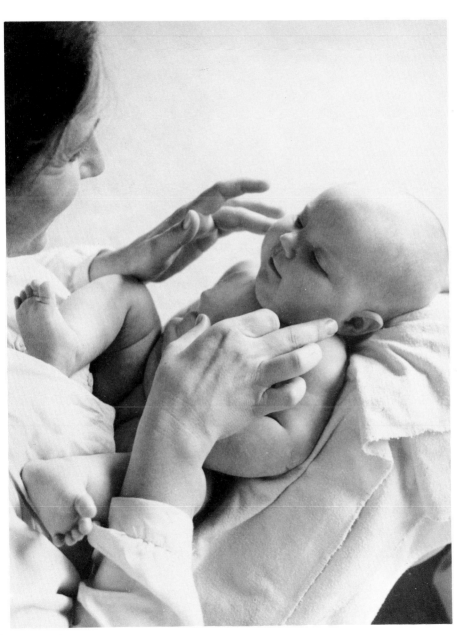

The Neck:
Very gently stroke the neck down from ears to shoulders and from chin to upper chest.

The Shoulders:
Stroke from the neck to the beginning of the arms.

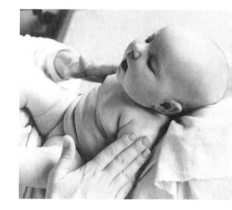

The Arms:
Stroke down from the shoulder to the fingertips. Then wrap your fingers and thumb around the arm and do a series of gentle squeezes, starting at the top of the arm and finishing at the wrist. Use alternate hands. Massage the wrist using thumb and forefinger.

The Hands:
Massage the hands, using the thumb for the palm, and the fingers for the back of the hand. Stroke each finger with the fingertips and thumb.

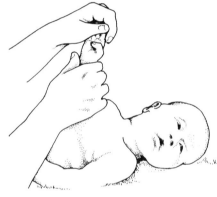

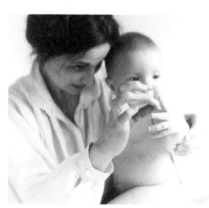

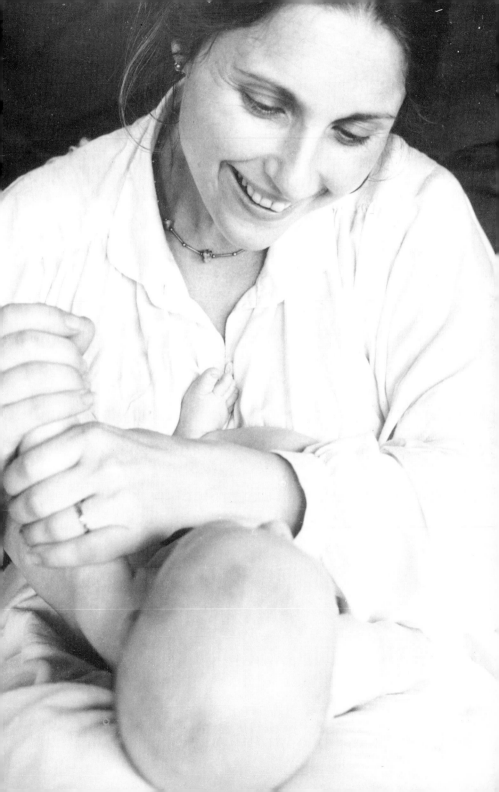

The Chest:

Using both hands, stroke the chest from the centre outwards to the sides of body, towards the back. Remember that the ribs curve and strokes should follow the spaces between the ribs (the intercostal spaces). Stroke the diaphragm along the edge of the rib cage.

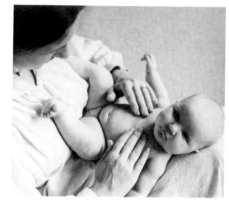

The Belly:

Use a clockwise circular massage around the umbilicus, in ever widening circles. Do this only after umbilical cord has separated (dropped off). This massage follows the course of the ascending, transverse and descending colon. Use the fingertips or the fingers and palms of hand.

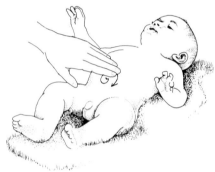

The Genitals:

Include in long strokes down the body, so that they are touched naturally as part of the whole body, not ignored, not accentuated.

The Legs:

Massage thighs, knees, shins and calves. Then gently squeeze from thigh to ankle (as with the arms).

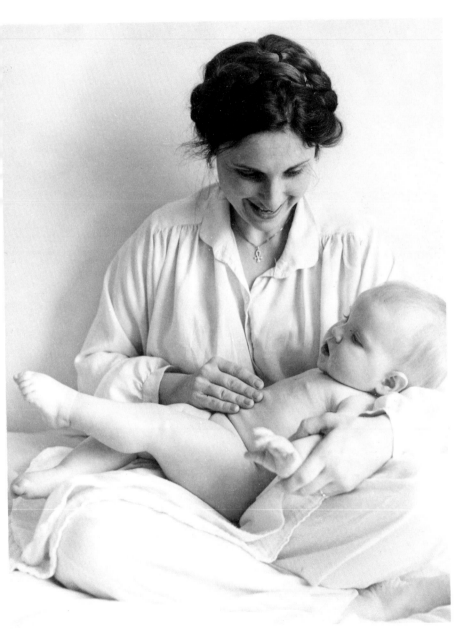

Feet and Ankles:

Massage the ankles, then in turn, supporting each ankle securely with one hand, use the thumb to massage the foot firmly from heel to toe along the sole of the foot. This is the firmest massage of the whole body. Stroke each toe, perhaps playing 'This Little Piggie'.

The Whole Front:

Using both hands, one for each half of the body, stroke from neck to toes including the arms and genitals on the way. This long light full body stroke can be repeated several times.

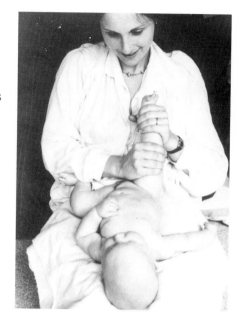

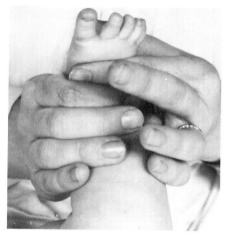

The Back of the Body
Turn baby over on to his belly and lay him across your thighs. Alternatively, if the baby is uncomfortable lying on his belly, hold him close to your body with his head just above your shoulder, so that his body is slightly curved. The back of the body can then be massaged, as he usually relaxes in this position. This is also a good position for the older baby having his first massage.

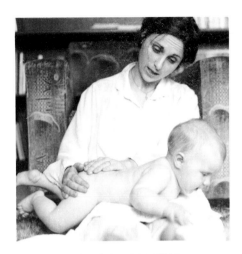

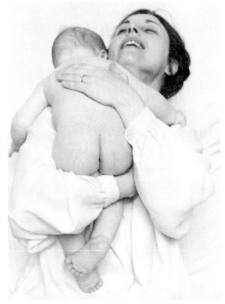

The Head:
With the fingers and palm of hand, stroke the crown of head down towards the neck until the bony ridge of the skull is reached (the occipital region).

The Neck:
From the top of the neck, using both hands simultaneously and with one or two fingers, gently massage the muscles at the side of the cervical spine, using a descending circular motion, to the base of the neck.

The Shoulders:
With the fingertips, gently move the muscles in a circular motion from the neck out towards the shoulders. Often your baby feels tense exactly where you feel tense, so if you are tense in the shoulders, give your baby some extra massage on his shoulders.

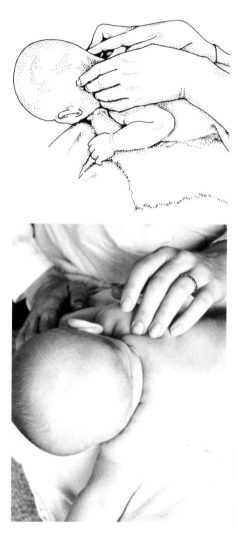

The Back:

With your hand stretched out across baby's back so that your hand is in contact with the whole width of his back, stroke down his back from neck to buttocks — including his buttocks. Then with the fingertips of both hands, lightly massage the muscles on either side of the spine, from neck to buttocks, again, using a descending circular movement.

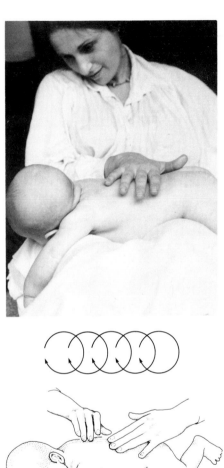

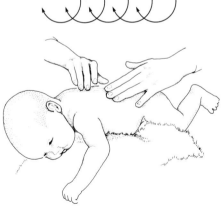

The Buttocks:
Jiggle the buttocks around playfully.

The Legs:
Give long strokes from the top of
the thighs to the toes.

Full Body Strokes:
From head to toe, starting on the
crown of the head, with the fingers
and the palm of the hand, give a
long, light, loving, sweeping stroke
down the back and finish beyond the
toes. Repeat several times.

You have come to the end of the
massage. Turn baby over, cover him
with a bunny rug and hold him for a
few minutes before dressing him.

Enjoy the moment!

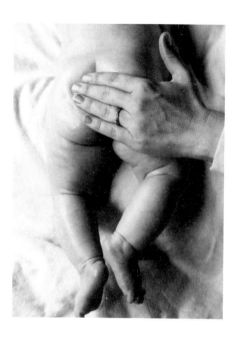

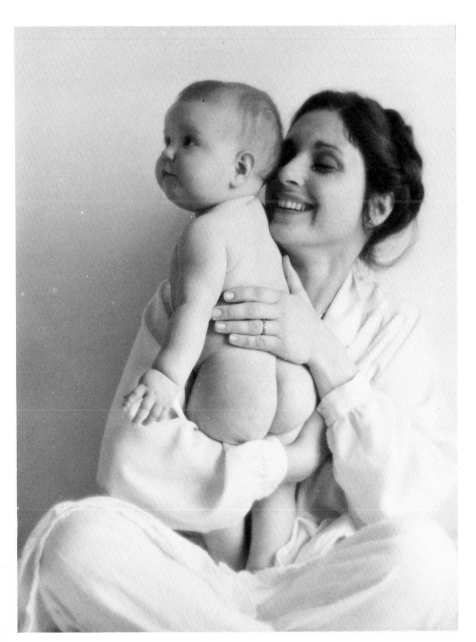

As your Baby Grows

The technique I have described is especially suitable for babies in the first nine months, but you can, of course, continue massaging your child effectively to any age. Toddlers, teenagers and adults can all benefit from massage. The same techniques can be used for older babies, though as they grow stronger you can massage more firmly. When introducing massage to older babies and children, choose a time when they are quiet, relaxed and receptive to stroking — perhaps at bath time, or when they are sitting on your knee listening to a story.

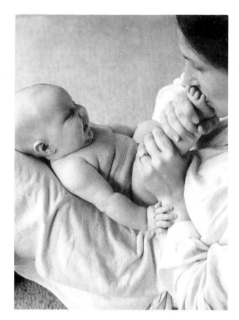

Creative Touches

You can experiment and find many other ways to touch and play that will delight you and your baby. Try licking, for example. This could be particulary soothing on the eyelids [see Chapter Five]. Kissing on the soles of the feet is another possibility. Tracing his body with your hair. Try Eskimo nose massage — use your imagination and your nose!

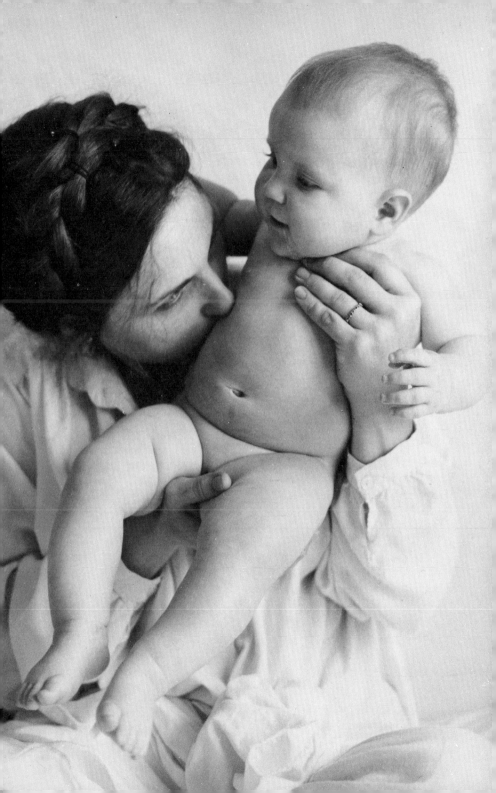

Massage for Babies with Special Needs

Massage can have a very beneficial effect on premature babies, emotionally disturbed infants, and babies with physical handicaps and those experiencing a development lag. It can also help prevent early negative experiences such as separation from their mothers, and painful nursing or medical procedures from adversely affecting their behaviour in later life.

Because of the calming effect of massage on mother and baby, as already noted I think that it is particularly useful for the unsettled, irritable, or 'colicky' baby, making the use of sedating drugs unnecessary. Some of these drugs are obtainable without prescription and are often used by mothers.

Blind or Deaf Babies
These babies would become more aware of their body shape and of themselves as a person.

Sandra Weiss, in her article, 'The Language of Touch' in **Nursing Research** (March/April, 1979) says:

> Jourard (1960) demonstrated that a person's perception of how much of the body is touched by others appears distinctly related to that person's positive evaluation of self.

> The literature consistently shows that an individual who receives body contact from others over most body areas, in contrast to only a few areas, generally feels more attractive, feels closer to other persons, possesses an accurate perception of the form and shape of his body and has a positive liking for himself.[5]

Elizabeth Panengyres (Physiotherapist-in-charge, Princess Margaret Hospital for Children, Perth, Western Australia) has observed a blind and deaf baby who loved a whole body massage, also a post-meningitis baby, twenty-three months old and ambulant, who enjoyed modified massage.

She also knows an eighteen months old post-meningitis, visually handicapped, quadriplegic boy who enjoys a face and leg massage, and she will gradually try to increase the area massaged as his sensitivity decreases.

Babies in the Pavlik Harness and the Dennis Brown Bar, used for Congenital Dislocation of the Hips
Over the past two years, five babies with congenital dislocation of the hip have attended my Infant Welfare Centre. They had the Pavlik Harness applied a few days after birth. This harness is kept on all the time, except when a new harness is fitted.

No bath is given to the baby during

e time he is in the harness (six to ne months, followed by the Dennis own Bar to approximately twelve onths). His face, limbs and bottom e washed, but his trunk is mostly vered with the straps of the rness, so skin stimulation in that ea is minimal.

aught these mothers to massage eir babies, using apricot or almond l, and sliding their hands nderneath the straps of the harness here possible. They reported that e babies really enjoyed their daily assage.

elieve that the sensory stimulation nich these babies received during assage, which otherwise they uld not have experienced, has en of tremendous benefit, and has ade it easier to adjust and catch up th their 'milestones', such as lling themselves up, when they are ally taken out of the harness and r.

dopted Babies
assage can be particularly useful in tablishing a bond between two rangers. Adoptive parents literally come parents overnight. As these rents miss out on feelings imulated by pregnancy and ildbirth, massaging their babies lps them to relate closely and gain nfidence in handling them.

a recent massage practice

session, I was thrilled to see, when an adoptive mother first started massaging her 'new' ten week old baby, the look of recognition and smile of acceptance that passed between them as they established eye contact, and the mother began to explore her baby through touch. This was a special moment for all three of us.

The Hypersensitive Baby
Occasionally, babies do not like to be touched at all. One mother of such a baby had this to say:

> Baby was extra sensitive. Nobody could nurse her but me, not even her father. She would panic if you took her anywhere there was a crowd. I never let anyone nurse her, and I didn't take her out unless it was absolutely necessary. Also, her daily massage helped her a lot. Now, at ten months, there is no sign at all of her extra sensitivity. No drugs or medication of any sort were used.

Massage was done on this baby daily — gradually building up to about twenty minutes — over a period of six months. The difference in this baby when I saw her and handled her at nine months was remarkable. She was smiling and happy, and certainly did not mind being touched.

45

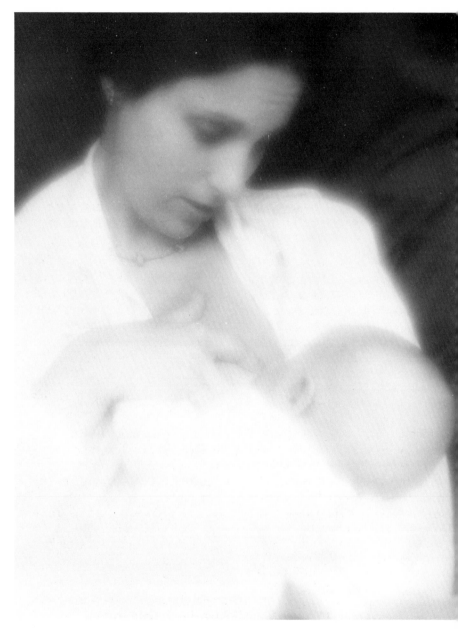

The Limp, Lethargic Baby
(Hyposensitive)

By contrast, such babies require much more stimulation before they respond. Such babies can be stimulated gently by massage, rather than relaxed by it. Various forms of light tickling, and a gentle but firmer pressure may be useful as they are massaged.

Premature Babies

These babies can gain great benefits from massage, as described by Eva Reich in Chapter Five.

If baby has not been given massage in hospital, the mother can start when she gets home. Often these babies need to learn that touch is pleasurable, since much that they have experienced at others' hands has hurt.

It is known that premature babies have reasonably well developed nervous systems which allow them to interact with their environment through touch, sight, sound, smell and taste, and that many of their inter-actions are not pleasant, but uncomfortable or painful because of procedures, monitoring, taking blood samples, etc.

Dr David Bannister [see Chapter Two] says of one small hospital: 'We certainly encourage gentle handling by the parents and sensory input through sound as well, by the parents making a tape of their voices and playing it inside the isolette. I certainly would be keen for massage to become a regular part of the programme for premature infants'.

Massage is also becoming a regular practice with premature babies in some major maternity hospitals throughout the country.

In such places, daily massage is given to unsettled, sensitive babies, or babies with a special problem.

It is valuable to help mothers who are apprehensive or nervous about their 'fragile' babies. They can watch a trained person do it and then do it themselves with this person standing by to help and give advice.

It can be started several weeks before the baby is due to go home. During this period the mothers are shown how to massage their babies and are given practice sessions.

An interesting link has been established with Tim Adair, who read my article on baby massage in the **Australian Nurses Journal.**[6] He is a paediatric physical therapist at the Research Medical Centre in Kansas City, U.S.A. He is working on a research programme of infant massage and stimulation with premature babies.

In October, 1980, he was asked by the Neonatologist at the Centre to begin instructing several mothers from the Special Care Nursery in the Massage/Stimulation (Rice) method for these babies. (Dr Ruth D. Rice researched and developed her 'Rice Infant Sensorimotor Stimulation' [RISS] technique in 1975. [See Chapter Seven.] This indicates a new approach in the U.S.A. to the care and development of the prematurely new-born baby.)

Some Specific Uses of Massage

Sudden Weaning or Difficult Weaning

A massage followed up by a bottle feed can be given in place of a breast feed if the baby is finding it hard to separate from his mother.

One mother, who had massaged her baby from a few months old, had difficulty in weaning her baby when he was nine months old. So, at his usual time for a breast feed (this was the feed at which he was difficult) she massaged his back, feet, or wherever he wanted to be massaged. She then gave him a bottle feed, which he took without refusing it or becoming upset. The mother continued doing this for one month, and now her baby enjoys his 7 p.m. bottle, and settles to sleep soon after taking it.

For the new baby having difficulty getting on the breast

It is helpful to stimulate the rooting reflex to achieve this. The rooting reflex is part of the normal baby's in-built reflex patterning. The baby opens his mouth and makes jaw and tongue movements which indicate searching. Gentle stroking from cheek to mouth towards the chin stimulates the rooting reflex, and the baby increases his searching, nuzzling and the opening of his mouth in his search for the nipple, which can then be put in his mouth. The sucking and swallowing reflexes follow on, completing the entire feeding act.

Teething

If he has been massaged at an earlier age, massage can be very effective in calming the teething baby.

Stroke the top of the head and the forehead to the ears, including the temple. Stroke from the base of the ears down to the base of the neck. Then stroke from the centre of the chin to the ears. Massaging the gums lightly can also be soothing. Mothers can use other body strokes that they know are soothing to baby.

Constipation

Abdominal massage can be very effective for babies with constipation. Use circular clockwise strokes around the umbilicus, thus following the course of the large bowel. [See Chapter Three — 'Technique'.]

Getting to Know Me

During the massage, advance the baby's awareness of his or her own body by touching his hand or foot to other parts of his body. For example, rubbing his foot along the length of his other leg, so he develops a feeling of the size, shape, texture, and special orientation of his body relative to other parts of him. Massage and self-exploration can be useful in preventing potential developmental and co-ordination problems.

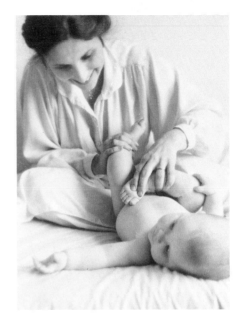

Birth Trauma in the New-Born

In this chapter, I have included contributions from other people. Dr Eva Reich comments about gentle bio-energetic massage therapy of the new-born. Bio-energetic massage stimulates the integration and flow of body energy. Ken Mellor's contribution includes the way he handled the birth trauma of his daughter immediately after birth. Jacqui Showell gives a short summary of her work and involvement with the irritable, 'colicky', super-sensitive baby. (These 'unsettled' babies often have a history of a difficult traumatic birth.)

Dr Eva Reich, M.D.

The following ideas about bio-energetic therapy of the new-born have been expressed by Dr Eva Reich in talks in Australia and other parts of the world. We have discussed these ideas together, and Dr Reich has demonstrated these principles in workshops which I have attended.

Primal therapy of babies at primal times seems to be the answer to the problems of human beings who suffer from pain related to their birth and the neonatal period.

I developed a 'butterfly touch' (a touch so light it does not remove the scales from a butterfly's wing), for the delicate massage of babies, in 1952, at the Harlem Hospital in New York City. It is based on the work of Wilhelm Reich, who first developed body therapy that he called bio-energetic medical orgone therapy. The technique is applied to the new-born for very brief periods of time, in a very lightly touching manner.

I think mothers, nurses and doctors, or anyone who has the care of new-born babies, could apply this massage technique if they understood the basic principle, which is that we work from the head towards the toes, very, very gently, that we try to flex the body into the attitude of orgasm reflex discovered by Dr Wilhelm Reich, by bringing forward the pelvis and the shoulders; that we understand something about allowing the chest to really breathe out in expiration, and we learn to know where the tensions of the new-borns are situated. When the baby responds, there must be something in the environment to return that response, otherwise baby has all reason to stay withdrawn.

Loving touch is important, and while doing the massage, tell the baby in a soft, gentle voice, that he is welcome in the world, that you are sorry if he had a hard birth and that it is very good that he is now here and that everything will be all right.

Ideally, the massage can be done in the delivery room for babies, especially for those who have had a hard birth. [See pages 52-56 as to how two parents managed the difficulties of their baby immediately after a hard home birth.] Massage can also be done in special care nurseries where babies are suffering various procedures, as babies there are only touched to 'do' a procedure for them, certainly not for the pleasure of touch.

Much body contact is the best natural therapy. The rocking motion of being in arms is excellent. A non-violent natural birth and as little anaesthetic as possible are also important.

Place the baby on his side to do the back, maintain eye contact, watch his facial expression, and work with the respirations of the anterior chest cage, aiding a wave of expiration to move towards the pelvis. This is a really good position, as the baby can be encouraged to flex.

The massage can easily be taught to the new mother. It is also important to work with the actual body tension and emotional reaction of the mother to the birth — her actual birth experience. I find the whole treatment works best when both the mother and the baby have a chance to express their emotions.

In talking about the small 1500 gram premature infant, Eva Reich says:

It is important to stroke and stimulate and massage and encourage the total expiration of the chest segment in the premature infant gently, because this will prevent the usual dependent pneumonias of the premature baby. In a series of babies that I did this with daily in Harlem Hospital in 1952, I found that none of them developed pneumonia, and neither did any of them die.

It is important to talk to the infant and tell him during the therapy that we understand that he is isolated, that he is having a difficult time in his infancy, that he is suffering various procedures, and that there will be a better time when he will go home to his mother. Treat him like a person who needs to understand what has happened to him.

It is very important that the person doing the massage loves the baby and that the touch be a loving touch.

I am convinced that the sleeping state — the withdrawal from the world of these premature infants — is an artifact of their environment, and in primal therapy people do re-experience the pain of their old isolation in the incubator.

I think all hospitals should welcome parents to be with their premature infants as much as possible, even if the infant is very tiny. (Incubators and 'Light Treatment Units' could be standing next to mother's bed as in the maternity section of the General Public Hospital at Pithiviers, in France, under Dr Michel Odent.)

I also believe that mothers of sick neo-nates have the right to be there.

Hospitals need to treat little babies as people.

Ken Mellor

Ken Mellor is a social worker in private practice in Melbourne, Australia. He is experienced in child development and family problem solving, and is also experienced in Neo-Reichian therapy.

Ken, his wife Paola, and their daughter Bianca, are the people in the beautiful photographs in this book.

When I heard Ken talking about Bianca's birth at home, I wanted to include something about it in my book. Ken agreed to write out an account of the birth and the following few months of Bianca's life. It is such an interesting and important example of bonding, dealing with birth trauma and a father's involvement, love and commitment in caring for his baby, that I have included the whole account.

Imprinting

Right from the time we discovered that Paola was pregnant, I was determined to be present at the birth of our baby. I wanted to bond with her so that she would be emotionally linked to me as well as to Paola. When discussing this with a knowledgeable friend early in the pregnancy, he said, 'You will probably not remember until the time, but do your best to have your upper body naked. That way, your baby will be able to smell your skin and feel what you are like much better than if you are dressed.' This made a lot of sense to me, and I determined to do it. I already had plans of my own and added this to them.

When Bianca arrived, I was duly dressed so that my chest was ready for direct skin contact with her. I was wearing a dressing gown that was easy to open at the front. After Paola had held Bianca on her stomach and we had stroked her gently for quite some time, and had put her to the breast, I took her. Before this, I had taken a fairly inactive role, as I did not want to interfere in the process taking place between them. However, at the point I took her, I wanted to be alone with her, and so be focused on her and she on me. So I stood up with her in my arms, held her out from me, and looked at her. She opened her eyes and gave me a long searching look of recognition and acceptance. I pulled her into my chest and held her closely to me. Then, as I had planned previously, I licked her thoroughly on her forehead, her eyes and her cheeks. I had planned to lick her face completely, but when it came to the point, I found it too awkward to do this while holding her upright against my chest. Another time, I would probably put her on something soft and bend over her to do it. In this way, I could have reached all parts of her face and other parts of her body quite easily.

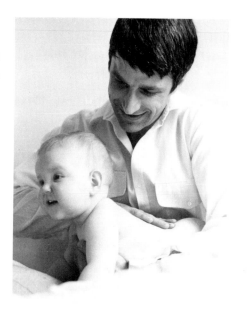

As I licked her, she seemed to relax; she seemed soothed. I was

53

pleasantly surprised at the taste. In advance, I had imagined that it might be a little unpleasant. But I found this not to be true. If anything, the taste was neutral. My main discomfort through the process was that I thought others in the room may have been watching and I was a little self-conscious about it. I have repeated the licking on several occasions since and have received a consistently pleasurable response from her. She seems to find it comforting. I felt a connection with her at birth and have continued to do so.

[See Ashley Montague's book, **Touching**.[7] All mammals lick their young with the tongue, except human beings, who touch gently with the fingers if not prevented from doing so.]

Dealing with birth trauma immediately after a birth

Bianca's head was born and it was immediately obvious that she was in trouble. The cord was around her neck and had stopped pulsing. The doctor and midwife went into action: quickly they unwound the cord and pulled her out. Her neck was slightly twisted in the process. As soon as she hit the doctor's hands, she drew breath and started to cry. I breathed a sigh of relief.

This would have been enough trauma for any baby to have to deal with, but it was not all. Throughout the birth, Paola had been in considerable pain. Added to this, she had breathed through the pushing contractions and prolonged the second stage to about one and a half hours. The result was that Bianca's head was very moulded. Some time after the birth, we noticed that there were three small bruises, almost abrasions, on the crown on her head. It was as though she had been scraped against something hard during the birth. This pressure was probably the cause of much of Paola's pain. In retrospect, it seems likely that she was in a transverse or posterior position and had sustained these injuries because of this. Meconium was on her crown when it was first visible, so she must have been in extreme distress from early in the labour.

From the moment of her birth, she whimpered and cried a little. She was not the peaceful, trauma free baby we had wanted to deliver. Nor did she seem able to settle. We did all the necessary things: bonding, putting her to the breast, massaging her gently and the like. Also, because the doctor needed the information for his records, we did things like weighing her; and I kept hoping that she would settle down. But she did not. Instead, as time passed, she became more and more distressed. Even a warm bath did not help settle her.

After about two hours or so, she was crying in great distress. It was then that I noticed that the bruises on her head had become much worse. They had combined to form one large bruise which extended over about one-third of her head, a very blue, very painful looking bruise. To relieve the pressure on this, we sat her upright in our arms and settled down to support her doing whatever she needed to do.

For about the next two and a half hours, she cried. She cried and cried, obviously in very great pain. Fortunately, we had many hours of sitting with grown-ups while they expressed the feelings — the pain — they had experienced during difficult births, and we knew two very important things. First, they had developed problems later as they had lacked support as babies while they expressed these feelings. Second, that the only way to express them seems to be to cry. So Paola and I simply held Bianca while she cried, occasionally taking turns when one of us needed a rest.

Quite quickly, it became apparent that she was working her way backwards through labour. Her crying spells came in bursts, roughly timed at two minutes apart, just as Paola's contractions had been for most of the labour. Presumably each contraction had brought more pain to Bianca as the pressure on her head was intensified. At the end of each bout of crying, during which she was in acute distress, sometimes coughing and struggling for breath, she would either become very peaceful and look around at us, or she would sleep peacefully for a few minutes. Each time she quietened down, especially after she had been going for a long time, I hoped against hope that she was through it all and would stop. But she had not finished and would soon become distressed again.

I was very aware that it was my distress I was wanting to alleviate by getting her to stop, and that she needed to cry or she would not be crying. This made it only marginally easier not to interfere. Many parents would need a great deal of support to feel secure enough not to interfere. Thinking that something was wrong, which it obviously would be, and that they should do something, as well as feeling their own distress, they might try and jiggle or cuddle their babies to stop them. They might also succeed. But if they did, then they would also succeed in getting their babies to hold onto the pain of birth and to the subsequent limitations that would go automatically with doing so. They would also stop an apparent miracle, the miracle of the human being's capacity to heal itself.

As we held her, talked to her, told her we loved her and that we were sorry that she was hurting, and that we wanted her to do what she needed to do, we watched this miracle take place. The bruising on her head went away, and so did the moulding. After each crying bout, there was a little less of each. Eventually, there was virtually none left, and she rested peacefully for some time.

In the succeeding three or four weeks, she cried fairly regularly in a similar manner at first. It was obvious at these times that she still had more pain to release. Her cry when doing this was quite distinctive. However, the frequency dropped over this period, so that from being about once a day to begin with, it became about once a week. After two months, it was only once a

fortnight; while now, at four and a half months, she seems to cry like this about once a month. Each crying spell has been from five minutes to one and a half hours.

The results have been worth it. There appear to be few if any residual effects of the birth. Also, Bianca impresses us and others as being contented, alert, very relaxed and very responsive. Above all, she seems to be completely secure both with us and with our friends; not a baby who is scared of people who are apparently neglecting her because they sit with her and let her cry when she is in pain from the past. Finally, when she cries now-a-days, we can tell what it is about. Almost always, it is about a here and now issue, and when, on the rare occasions, it is not, we can tell by the quality of her cry and know that the best thing to do is to hold her while she cries it out. I think that leaving her to do this alone, either earlier on or now, would have been, and still is, a very bad idea.

Jacqui Showell

Jacqui Showell is a physiotherapist, working in Adelaide with the Mothers and Babies Health Association. She is particularly involved with the irritable 'colicky' baby under four months, whom she

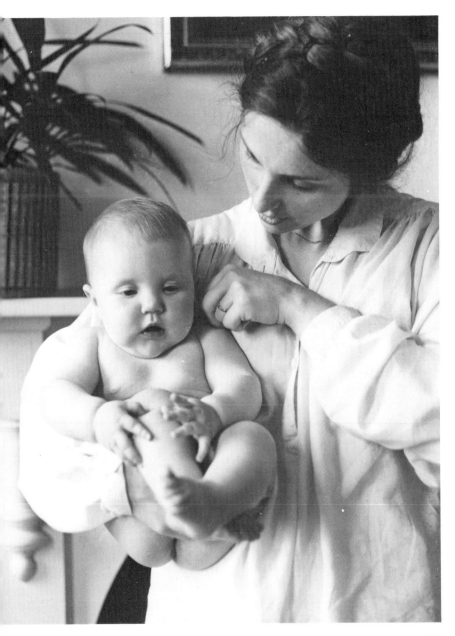

feels is often super-sensitive to the environment and his own body. Jacqui says about her work:

I use massage in conjunction with handling techniques to give some continuation of the familiar uterine world. Included are handling the babe in flexion (similar to the usual foetal position), maximum body contact, slow, firm cushioned movements, deep floaty baths, sheep skins to sleep on, and being carried as much as possible in a sling on the parent's body. The parents may also attend my relaxation and discussion group and, where possible, receive some massage from me — for their relaxation, to get some nurturing and energy, and to experience what they will give their babies.

The very young babies are always held in flexion, and they are massaged while they are in this flexed foetal position. Gradually they are helped to cope with more extended postures.

My techniques are adapted from my physiotherapy training, Gerda Boyesen's 'bioenergy massage', as taught in her institute in London, and other forms of healing such as acupressure. However, most of my learning has been from babies and their

mothers over a three year period of intuitive exploration.

The flexed position, as illustrated on page 57 is a useful way to hold baby if he is upset and arching his back. The position of flexion relaxes his abdominal muscles, calms him down, and gives you a free hand to answer the telephone, for example.

Another flexed position is with the baby curled up in the semi-foetal position on his side, his head forward on his chest and his knees drawn up to his belly. This is a good position in which to massage the premature baby.

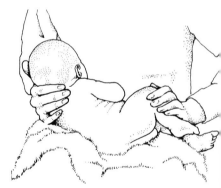

Nurturing and Support for Parents

I have been emphasising the baby's needs for loving touching, but in this chapter I now turn to the equally important subject of meeting the needs of the parents. The emotions and behaviour of the parents and that of the baby have a strong influence on each other, so it is vital that the parents, as well as the baby, have their needs adequately met.

The parents who are emotionally and physically well nourished are better able to provide the care needed for their baby's full development. They will also find it easier to cope with day-to-day management of the baby. Raw nerves and reliance on tranquillisers or stimulants can thus be lessened or eliminated.

Nurturing is being cared for, nourished, fed.

We all need nurturing, particularly at times when we have to give out a lot to others. Massage is an important and pleasurable way of receiving nurturing.

Some of the ways of being nurtured by others — partner, family or friends — are by having a foot, head or neck and shoulders massage, or a full body massage.

Think back to when you were a child. In what ways were you nurtured then. Think of things that made you feel good, such as sitting on your father's knee and being cuddled, having your hair washed or brushed, or having your back scratched or rubbed. Do you ask your partner to nurture you in any of these or other ways now?

Self-Nurturing
What is a self-nurturing experience for you? A bubble bath? An early night? An unhurried nourishing meal? Time to paint, enjoy music, or read a book? Time to just be? Make time for some self-nourishment, today — no matter how brief.

Support Systems
Because the 'extended family' (more than two generations living together or nearby) seems to be diminishing in significance in our society today, it is important that parents with young children become aware of the supporting groups and services that are available, and learn how to use them. Examples include groups of nursing mothers and child-minding groups. Also, a circle of supporting friends, maybe including 'foster-grandparents' can be an enriching experience for parents, children and friends, and can make the task of parenting easier to cope with.

Feelings
When a new baby arrives in the family, particularly if it is a first child, many new and often unexpected stresses and tensions are added to the parents' lives, as changes in their

relationships and routine occur. Previously buried feelings may surface in ways the parents find hard to explain.

At the time of the actual birth, the atmosphere of excitement, anticipation and, perhaps, fear, with the rhythmic contractions of the mother and then with the baby appearing, may cause many of those observing to be put in contact with their own internal feelings of being a baby and being born. These sensations can be very strong, and occasionally a person witnessing a birth may start to experience being confined and short of breath, to feel anger at the way the medical staff are treating the baby, or to feel fear of any pain being experienced. But they may not be aware of why they are experiencing such strong feelings. (This may explain why some hospital staff are sometimes very anxious to administer drugs to the mother as she goes into strong labour — feeling panic and distress arising as they start to contact the memory of their own painful birth.) An attempt by someone to suppress any manifestation of birth feelings in someone else is probably an attempt to suppress it in themselves.

Parents also often have feelings of great joy and elation following child-birth, and sometimes experience a release of spiritual energy immediately after, and for several weeks after, the birth of their baby. This is a happy, important time in the lives of parents, grand-parents, siblings and friends.

Flow with the energy of the feelings you have, so that the energy is supporting instead of conflicting; laugh if you are happy, cuddle if you are loving, cry if you are sad, go to another room and shout if you are angry or scared. Physically expressing strong feelings provides a safe outlet, thus avoiding a build up of tension in our bodies.

Changes and Adjustments
With the addition of a baby to their lives, parents find that there are changes in their relationship and adjustments to be made.

The husband and wife change from being a care-free couple, usually with two pay packets and often living a full life with many outside interests, to parents with the constant responsibility of caring for their baby, and less money to live on. Adjusting as parents is often difficult, although to some couples it comes naturally. In any case, with patience, understanding, love and sharing, successful adjustment can be achieved.

Your relationship as a couple is important, so make time to spend with each other at home. Share your life. Get a baby-sitter occasionally to mind baby (grand-parents usually enjoy this job), and have a night out together.

For the mother, it often means being no longer in the workforce. This can involve loss of friends, loss of identity, loss of structure and loss of financial independence, resulting in feelings of grief. This loss of identity stems from being a capable, efficient and important person in her occupation and then, after the arrival of the baby, becoming a mother and being referred to as a 'housewife' with little or no status. This often has a devastating effect on a woman, especially if she previously had an interesting career. She is sometimes lonely and isolated, relying on her husband to meet most of her emotional needs, and may develop the 'suburban neurosis syndrome'.

Also, a mother who has been brought up in a nuclear family often has no experience of handling small babies, and as a result is often anxious and scared about specific things, and may be generally confused and lacking confidence. Nurturing from her partner, family and friends will help this mother to deal with her scared feelings; support and information as she learns to use it will help her with her confusion and lack of confidence. To be held, cuddled or caressed when feeling scared is comforting and reassuring.

Adjusting to the Baby

It takes time to get to know your baby. Take the time to do this. You may need to learn to accept being a parent and the changes it brings. Knowing that this takes time may help you to be at peace with yourself. This can be an exciting and rewarding time of your life. Being available to your baby will help you discover parenting as an on-going living experience. Enjoy as much of it as you can and practise being a creative parent.

Dr David Bannister has this to say:

One of the things I find that is very important is the changes or adjustments parents have to make especially with their first baby.

They can be told and warned, but it still comes as a shock to a lot of parents, particularly the first few weeks with a new creature they know nothing or very little about. I tell them that having babies is a lottery — you do not know what temperamental characteristics they have inherited from the parents, or what are their own entirely different ones. It takes time, sometimes, to get to know this new person, and it can be a very stressful time for **all**. It can also be fun and absorbing getting to know your own baby, but parents need to be given 'permission' to experiment, to find out their baby's likes and dislikes and not necessarily stick to rigid schedules.

Where we, as health professionals, all too often go wrong, is in giving directions to parents, rather than advice or suggestions that might or might not work. We should be encouraging the parents to find out for themselves, i.e. develop their **own** parenting skills, rather than become dependent on others for what to do.

Stress
Hans Selye, in his book, **Stress Without Distress,** says:

Stress is the non-specific response of the body to any demands made on it — when we say someone is under stress, we usually mean excessive stress or distress.[8]

Stress can be produced from a pleasant or unpleasant experience. How we react to stress or distress is what counts.

At childbirth and for about six to eight weeks after, mothers and fathers can be under excessive stress, especially if the baby cries more often than usual and both parents do not get enough sleep.

One important way of dealing with stress is to find the cause and make some changes.

Mothers' Special Needs
If the mother is feeling exhausted and tired, perhaps it could be arranged for a relative or friend to help with the housework, or to get in the Council Home Help if available. Usually this is available at a reasonable charge, for at least three weeks after the mother gets home from hospital. This could be a good 'present' to give the new mother, allowing her to have some time to herself.

If the situation warrants it, it might be arranged for someone to sit up with the new mother during the night feed for moral support, or arranged for the husband or grandparent to give the baby the night feed for a few nights so that the mother can have a longer sleep.

If the baby is breast fed, maybe enough milk can be expressed during the day for a night feed. Lactation sometimes fails if the mother becomes too exhausted through lack of sleep. Having a sleep during the day or going back to bed after the early morning feeding, are also ways of getting more rest, and helping to maintain the milk supply.

As well as being tired through lack of sleep, for the first few weeks after childbirth, mothers are often physically and emotionally depleted. What they are likely to need is caressing and energising through loving touch. As sexual intercourse is generally not resumed until after bleeding has stopped, this closeness and body contact is often missing. Of course, couples can learn ways of sexually pleasuring each other without genital contact.

Massage can be a non-sexual nuturing and energising experience for a new mother, renewing her energy level and so enabling her to meet the baby's need for emotional and physical nourishment. A back and shoulder massage can be given to the mother while she is sitting comfortably in a bean bag, perhaps while nursing or feeding the baby, or maybe watching T.V., and her husband can sit behind her to give the massage. More generally, mothers could ask husbands, partners, family or friends for some massage, or a hug, or a caress when they are tired, or when they feel like being nurtured.

I believe that a full body massage given to mothers on the second or third day after child-birth and frequently during the next six weeks, could help prevent post-natal depression, as mothers themselves often feel the need to be held and caressed during this time.

Physical Benefits for Mothers from Massage

Massage dilates the blood vessels, improving the circulation and relieving congestion throughout the body.

Massage relaxes muscle spasms and relieves tension.

Massage increases the blood supply and nutrition to muscles without adding to their load of toxic lactic acid. (Lactic acid is a by-product of muscular activity, produced when insufficient oxygen is present in the muscular tissue to prevent its formation. It is present in tired or sore muscles.) Massage thus helps to prevent the build-up of harmful 'fatigue' products resulting from strenuous exercise or injury.

Massage helps you to feel good.

In Malaysia, mothers are massaged on their second or third day after the birth of their baby, and then every day for six weeks. The massage is usually done by the mother, mother-in-law, or even the grand-mother. Australian women I have spoken to about this Malaysian custom respond with, 'Wow! Wouldn't that be wonderful'.

Ashley Montague, in his book, **Touching**,[9] quotes Reva Rubin as saying that meaningful touch administered during labour, actual birth and immediately after birth, influences the mother towards a more effective use of her hands, whereas remote, impersonal contact induces similar attitudes towards contact with her baby. Montague suggests that it may be a good idea for the husband to caress his wife's body 'during pregnancy, labour and after the birth of the baby'.

In some Melbourne hospitals, abdominal massage is given to mothers after child-birth by the physiotherapist. Why not back, or indeed a full body massage?

It seems to me that home deliveries provide very well for the nuturing needs of mothers and fathers. As well as the doctor and midwife, there can be one or two support people, usually close friends or relatives, and the mother can receive a lot of physical contact and strokes from her husband and the support people, both during labour and after the baby has been born. Jealousy in siblings is generally unknown when they are part of the birth experience.

General Support
After the birth of a baby, whether at home or in hospital, support, nurturing and help for baby, mother and father and other children, are most important. Family and friends usually supply this support. However, where young families are isolated from their parents, people working with young families professionally, such as the Royal District Nursing Service Nurses and Infant Welfare Nurses, give very valuable support. The Nursing Mothers' Association is also very supportive and can provide contacts so that people can help each other.

In the first few weeks after the baby is born, it is important that the new mother gets out of the house with the baby and has a break from the 'at home' feeding, bathing, nappy washing routine. Many Infant Welfare Centres in Victoria have New Mothers Groups where such mothers can talk about their problems and worries over a cup of tea, and learn the next stages of growth and development of their babies and parenting skills, including baby massage, from the Maternal and Child Health Nurse.

In my experience, these young mothers have a great need to talk about what is happening with them and their babies, and it often helps to know that other mothers have problems and feelings similar to their own. After six weeks, when the groups that I conduct finish, these mothers often continue meeting in their own homes as well as meeting again at the Health Centre with me at three monthly intervals. Firm supporting friendships are made, and as the babies become older, play groups are formed.

Many new parents, especially mothers, resist asking for help, believing that they should be able to cope with their baby and home, that if in fact they cannot manage by themselves, they are failures as mothers. But, the real fact is that it is difficult for a mother to do all the caring for a baby and herself without help from her husband, family or friends. If isolation affects the mother in a negative way, this feeling is transferred to the baby. Babies benefit from extra contact with others, rather than just the mother and father.

I suggest that you ask for and accept help, and share your baby with others. It is all right to be helped!

Fathers' Special Needs.

The family with a young baby can be seen as an energy circuit. There is the young baby needing energy, but the mother at this stage is often low in energy due to fatigue and the constant demands of her new-born baby. The father, who is stimulated by his activities outside the family, can be seen as a battery supplying energy to the mother and through her to the baby. The baby at this stage still belongs in the mother's energy field; that is, he still has a close energy link with his mother. The mother is the most important person in the baby's life. Fathers may experience themselves providing energy for everyone for some time — and they need replenishing, too.

This does not mean that fathers only have contact with their baby through the mother. In fact, it is important that they have direct contact with baby from birth onwards and so build up a warm loving relationship with their child. Besides cuddling and holding the baby, father can feed the baby if bottle fed, bathe the baby or have a bath with baby — and massage the baby. Fathers who have been present at the birth of their child, usually become more involved in the care of their baby, feel part of the whole birth experience and feel closer to their child.

If a father has paternity leave or a week off work when his wife comes home with the new baby, this gives him an opportunity to get to know the new baby and give practical support and help to his wife. If there is a toddler in the family, the father could spend a lot of time with him, thus helping to eliminate some of the jealous feelings the toddler may have towards the new baby, and the mother can then give less divided attention to the new baby.

The father is a very important member of the family, but with the mother's time being mostly taken up with the care of the new baby, leaving little time or energy to share with her husband, he may feel neglected. Also, the temporary cessation of sexual intercourse with his wife could result in him feeling the lack of intimate, pleasurable touching and caressing. However, this need not be the case if this couple had learned to relate non-sexually through close body contact and pleasurable touching without always having sexual intercourse or genital contact. This subject is sensitively explored in Helen Kaplan's book, **The New Sex Therapy.**[10] A sensitive sensuous massage is one way of experiencing this.

I have talked to fathers about their needs and suggested that they have a weekly body massage from a caring person. While they agree that this is a good idea, they think it would be difficult to find such a masseur; the Gym. type football masseur or the massage parlour masseuse being quite unsuitable. However, there are some caring masseurs, and maybe they could advertise as such.

I have been emphasising problems, but I recognise that the new baby also brings with him or her many joys and satisfactions, and that parents, as well as coping with the distresses, can have fun with their baby and experience pleasure and

pride in nurturing their child.

A **conscious** awareness of your own needs and the needs of others, makes it possible for the whole family to co-operate in getting their needs met in a positive way.

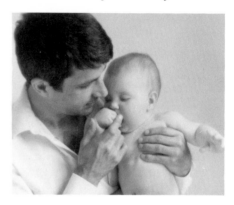

Baby Massage in Other Cultures

In this chapter I want to show that older cultures recognise the value of baby massage and close body contact; for example, by mothers using baby massage as a natural custom in the daily care of their infants and by constantly carrying babies close to their bodies. It is, however, not intended as a complete world-wide review of these practices.

Modern Western civilisation is only recently re-discovering these practices and finding scientific reasons for accepting them. It is sad that in our Western society some of us have to learn **how** to touch and **be** touched lovingly. It is not this way in many cultures. For example, skin and body contact form an important part of parenting in many parts of Nigeria, Uganda, India, Bali, Venezeula, Fiji and New Guinea.

Many women in tribal, nomadic, urban or rural environments carry on their usual work with their babies contentedly supported in slings. Clothing is often adapted into slings for this purpose. These babies, close to their mothers' bodies, experience a rocking, rhythmical movement which can stimulate their motor and intellectual development.

Nigeria

Conversation with Aisha Abubaker, a mother and midwifery nurse educator from Nigeria, 1980:

Babies are massaged from birth until they are twelve months old, and it is usual for most mothers to massage their babies. This is a very old custom which is passed on from mother to daughter, and has now become part of their child care routine. Commonly, the baby is bathed twice a day, at 7 a.m. and 5 p.m., and then massaged with olive oil. Firm strokes are used. During the massage, the mother's hands are warmed several times by the charcoal fire or a heater.

After six weeks, the baby is likely to be massaged in a sitting position, helping to strengthen his back muscles in readiness to sit up alone.

Most mothers have their baby at home, or, if they enter hospital, tend to stay for only six hours. Midwives practice in the community and also deliver babies in hospitals unless there are complications.

Baby is carried on the mother's back, secured with the mother's skirt — a long length of material which doubles as a baby sling and a skirt. A small towel or baby shawl is sometimes tied around the waist and under the baby's buttocks for added security.

For six weeks after childbirth, the practice is for the mother just to care for herself and the new baby. Other women in the family, usually the baby's grandmother, take over the work normally done by the mother. The new mother generally stays in her mother's house if they live nearby, and the husband visits her briefly each day. He is not very involved, as having babies is 'women's business'.

Uganda

Joseph Chilton Pearce, in **Magical Child**[11], writes about the research of Marcelle Gerber, who in 1956, travelled to Africa to study the effects of malnutrition on infant and child intelligence. He says that Marcelle Gerber, in Uganda, discovered that the Ugandan children were the most intelligent and advanced she had observed anywhere. Is is significant that the children were delivered at home, usually by the mother herself; or if she was on the move, out in the bush. Separation, mother from child, did not occur. The mother massaged, caressed, fondled and sang to her baby constantly from birth. Carried in a sling, the baby was next to her bare breast and fed according to its own needs. The baby and mother slept together. These Ugandan babies were alert, happy and calm, and were awake longer than is usual. Bonding with their mothers was strong, with the mothers anticipating their babies' needs before they needed to cry for attention. For the first four years of life, Gerber noticed a superior intellectual development.

India

Frederick Leboyer, in his beautiful book, **Loving Hands**[12], shows the traditional art of Indian massage which originated in South India, and is passed down from mother to daughter.

Throughout most of India, babies are regularly massaged from the age of about one month to six months. In the winter, diluted mustard oil is used, and in the summer, coconut oil.

Leboyer says:

> It is a sacred art in the true sense, since it is concerned with babies, with the renewal of life.

Bali

Speaking to a Balinese mother, I learned that in Bali babies are handled and stroked to comfort them. A child born in Bali is believed to have just emerged into this life from a spiritual realm, and is regarded as holy. For about two years, he is not permitted to touch the impure earth, and is carried about by his mother or by older children, either in their arms or on their hips.

The Indonesian mother carries her child in a length of cloth known as a 'Kain Panjang', wrapped around her body. The child is carried in front for ready access to breast milk. As the child grows larger, he is carried on the side of the woman's body, still within reach of his food. Only after weaning, is the child located on the mother's back.

There is a strong folk tradition of massage in Bali. 'Every single person' can do some massage, as many tourists have discovered.

If a baby in Bali has a pain in the gut, the spirit doctor is called in. He massages the baby's belly with a mixture of coconut oil, a crushed, small, red onion and salt. The massage lasts for about fifteen minutes. The baby is usually not fed for several hours, or until after he has used his bowels.

Fiji
Most Fijian mothers massage their babies with coconut oil following their daily bath. Massage is often given at night to settle the baby and to ensure that he sleeps well. Babies are carried close to the body in a sling fashioned from the mother's skirt.

New Guinea
In Wewak, New Guinea, the baby is carried in a 'bilum' string carrier, with the handle as a band around the forehead of the mother, the baby resting on the mother's bare back. **Pikinini i cri long skin belong mama** is a common Pidgin-English remark heard when a baby cries, meaning: 'The baby is crying to be close to his mother's skin'. Literally, 'skin to skin'. For feasts and special occasions babies, from one month of age, are rubbed or 'greased' with coconut oil.

New Zealand
The Maori
Christone Macdonald, in her, **Medicines of the Maori**[13], says:

> On the east coast the baby was covered with Muka scraping, the silky floss from the inner leaf of the flax. This they called **kukukuku**.

> In olden times, this was the covering for the first two or three weeks of life. Morning and evening, this was removed, the baby washed, and then gently massaged, the mother using a little warm oil (usually from the titoki). The baby was again covered tightly in fresh warm leaves, the moss and cape . . .

> Massage was considered highly important and was continued for

several years, the mothers using different movements of their hands. Knees and ankles received special attention, so that these joints would always be supple.

> Massage the legs of your daughter,
> So she will walk with grace
> Across the plains **(maraes)** of Poverty Bay.
>
> Dr T. Wirepa[14]

Maori women today have much body contact with their babies and frequently stroke them.

Venezuela

In her excellent book, **The Continuum Concept**[15], Jean Liedloff describes her experiences with the Yequana Indians in Venezuela.

She discovered that these people make use of the principle of energy exchange [See Chapter Two] between infant and caretaker when the infant is kept in close contact with the body of the caretaker With close body contact, the baby's body energies are kept in a state of balance. The result is a happier, healthier child.

Russia

The following report is by Ross G. Mitchell:

Soviet scientists believe that exercises and massages promote the formation of new communications within the central nervous system and the development of greater motor potentialities in consequence.

Whatever the theoretical basis for massage, (many) mothers and doctors in the Soviet Union are convinced that it makes the body and limbs more supple, strengthens and tones the muscles and skin, and generally increases the infants' well-being.

In the Soviet Union, it is an accepted and . . . practised part of child care. These mothers are taught to massage and exercise their infants from the first few days of life, and prominence is given to illustrations and descriptions of the technique in books and films on mothercraft. In residential homes for children much staff time is devoted to massage. Paediatricians and other health workers are sure of its value and counter the question: 'Why do you do it?' with 'Why don't you?'

Although massaging healthy babies is a custom virtually unknown in Western countries, except in immigrant communities, it is common in some parts of Africa and Asia.

... Can a technique practised by millions of mothers be so unimportant?[16]

The United States of America
In the U.S.A. in 1975 the (RICE) Rice Sensorimotor Stimulation technique was developed and researched by Dr Ruth D. Rice[17]. This consisted of stroking, massaging and rocking and is being accepted as a 'new' technique to enhance the care and development of premature babies.

It was found that in the babies who received 'The Loving Touch', as her technique is now called, there was a significantly greater neurological development, greater weight gain and a higher score in mental functioning than the babies receiving routine care.

[See Chapter Five] for Dr Eva Reich's work at the Harlem Hospital, New York in 1952.

Massage in an expression of love through loving caring touch.

References

1 Frederick Leboyer, **Birth Without Violence**, Fontana, U.K., 1977.
2 Marshall H. Klaus & John H. Kennell, **Maternal-Infant Bonding**, The C. V. Mosby Company, St. Louis, U.S.A., 1976.
3 Ashley Montague, **Touching**, Harper & Row, New York, N.Y., Second Edition, 1978.
4 Jean Liedloff, **The Continuum Concept**, First Futura Publications, London, 1976.
5 Sandra Weiss, 'The Language of Touch' in **Nursing Research**, March/April, 1979.
6 A. D. Auckett, S.R.N., 'Baby Massage: An Alternative to Drugs', in **The Australian Nurses' Journal**, November, 1979, Melbourne.
7 Montague, op. cit.
8 Hans Selye, **Stress Without Distress**, Hodder & Stoughton, Great Britain, 1975.
9 Montague, op. cit.
10 Helen Singer Kaplan, M.D., **The New Sex Therapy**, Ballier Tindale, London, 1974.
11 Joseph Chilton Pearce, **Magical Child**, Paladin Books, Frogmore, St. Albans, U.K., 1979.
12 Leboyer, id., **Loving Hands**, William Collins, London, 1977.
13 Christine Macdonald, **Medicines of the Maori**, William Collins, Auckland, N.Z., 1973.
14 T. Wirepa, (Dr), taken from a proverb in an article on the genealogical origin of his wife in **Te Toa Takati Magazine**, 1925-26, N.Z.
15 Liedloff, loc. cit.
16 Ross G. Mitchell, (1976) 'Is Kneading Needed?' in **Developmental Medical Child Neurology**, 18, 1-2.
17 Ruth D. Rice, Ph.D., 'The Rice Infant Sensorimotor Stimulation', in **The National Foundation, March of Dimes, 1979**, Newborn Behavioural Organization, Nursing Research and Implications, Allan Liss, Publisher, 1980.

Bibliography

Kaplan, Helen Singer, M.D., **The New Sex Therapy**, Ballier Tindale, London, 1974.

Klaus, Marshall H. & Kennell, John H., **Maternal-Infant Bonding**, The C. V. Mosby Company, St. Louis, U.S.A., 1976.

Leboyer, Frederick, **Birth Without Violence**, Fontana, U.K., 1977.

Leboyer, id., **Loving Hands**, William Collins, London, 1977.

Liedloff, Jean, **The Continuum Concept**, First Futura Publications, London, 1976.

Macdonald, Christine, **Medicines of the Maori**, William Collins, Auckland, N.Z., 1973.

Montague, Ashley, **Touching**, Harper & Row, New York, N.Y., Second Edition, 1978.

Pearce, Joseph Chilton, **Magical Child**, Paladin Books, Frogmore, St. Albans, U.K., 1979.

Selye, Hans, **Stress Without Distress**, Hodder & Stoughton, Great Britain, 1975.

Index